Give Her Multiple Big-O As Often As You Want

87 Simple Tips & Tricks to Giving a Woman Full-Body, Mind-Blowing, Explosive Climax Again and Again

Natalie Robinson

Copyright© 2018 by Natalie Robinson

Give Her Multiple Big-O As Often As You Want

Copyright© 2018 Natalie Robinson
All Rights Reserved.

Warning: The unauthorized reproduction or distribution of this copyrighted work is illegal. No part of this book may be scanned, uploaded or distributed via internet or other means, electronic or print without the author's permission. Criminal copyright infringement without monetary gain is investigated by the FBI and is punishable by up to 5 years in federal prison and a fine of $250,000. (http://www.fbi.gov/ipr/). Please purchase only authorized electronic or print editions and do not participate in or encourage the electronic piracy of copyrighted material.

Publisher: Enlightened Publishing

ISBN-13: 978-1986867269

ISBN-10: 1986867269

Disclaimer

The Publisher has strived to be as accurate and complete as possible in the creation of this book. While all attempts have been made to verify information provided in this publication, the Publisher assumes no responsibility for errors, omissions, or contrary interpretation of the subject matter herein. Any perceived slights of specific persons, peoples, or organizations are unintentional.

This book is not intended for use as a source of legal, business, accounting or financial advice. All readers are advised to seek services of competent professionals in the legal, business, accounting, and finance fields.

The information in this book is not intended or implied to be a substitute for professional medical advice, diagnosis or treatment. All content contained in this book is for general information purposes only. Always consult your healthcare provider before carrying on any health program.

Table of Contents

Introduction 3

Chapter 1: What is an Orgasm Anyway? 5

Chapter 2: Her Non-Sexual Erogenous Zones 11

Chapter 3: Inside the Vagina 23

Chapter 4: The Clitoris—How Find the Hot Spot 31

    Fingering Techniques 32

    Oral Sex Techniques 37

Chapter 5: The G-Spot—Myths and Facts about the Big Squirt 43

Chapter 6: The U-Spot, A-Spot, P-Spot and Deep Spot 51

    The U-Spot 51

    The A-Spot 52

    The P-Spot and Deep Spot 54

Chapter 7: The Elusive Mental Orgasm.......... 59

Chapter 8: Masturbation—Back to School, Folks!............... 67

    Steps of Learning the Female Orgasm (for Women) 70

    Masturbation Techniques 71

Chapter 9: Fetish Sex and Eroticism — To Boldly Go Where Few Men Have Gone Before 79

    The Key to Heightening Orgasmic Potential..................... 80

    Fetishism and BDSM 85

Chapter 10: How to be a Considerate Lover. 89

    How to be a Dominant Lover or a Horny Submissive 92

Chapter 11: The Most Common Mistakes Guys Make in Bed 95

Chapter 12: Cures for Performance Anxiety and Anorgasmia 101

Conclusion 105

Introduction

The Female Orgasm is indeed the new age version of the Holy Grail, a mysterious event that seems to boggle our imagination, challenge a man's ego, and sometimes elude us in much the way as a secret cave.

But wait! How about all that stuff I see in erotica books and Internet porn? Those guys make it look easy. So it should be just that easy, right?

And that's why we have so many real world sex problems. Because we all sort of think, yeah orgasms should be like that. So why isn't it working just like that?

Probably because studying erotica in place of education is sort of like getting your history lesson from, well, a Hentai cartoon.

- Real sex is not exaggerated.

- Real orgasms are not mechanical.

- Really good, awesome and out of this world sex takes practice, patience and strategizing rather than just wishing it to be.

It's like the old expression goes – if you build it they will come. Or in this case, if you really work at it, she will *come*.

This book is not going to tell you how it "should" happen, or how you wish it could happen—but rather how realistically you're going to either give a woman an orgasm, if you're a man, or bring yourself to orgasm with a lover, if you're a woman.

We're going to analyze the anatomy, the emotional complexity and the "social obligation" of all things orgasm over the course of 87 tips and 12 chapters.

By the end of the book, you're going to have your PhD in Orgasmology, or at least the equivalent of it. And the proof will be in those authentic moans of ecstasy, never more unrestrained, raw and amazing.

So let's get started in discussing the basics first…just what is an orgasm, anyway?

Chapter 1: What is an Orgasm Anyway?

An orgasm should be easy to define, right? It's when a woman loses all control and starts scream and shaking like the latest victim of *The Walking Dead*.

That's your first mistake. An orgasm doesn't actually "look" like anything specific, since it's a highly individual process. Men and women orgasm in different ways, according to different timetables and physical-emotional needs, and no one really orgasms in exactly the same way.

An orgasm is defined as a sexual climax and the sudden discharge of accumulated sexual arousal during the sexual response cycle.

Now it is true that some physical reactions do seem predictable when someone orgasms. For instance, both men and women feel the following when an honest to goodness orgasm happens:

- Feelings of euphoria
- Pulsating and "contracting" sensations in the genitals and perhaps over the "whole body"
- Flexing and relaxing muscles
- Aural undulations (or you know, the "oh oh oh!" we all know and love)

Of course, the female orgasm is slightly more complicated than the male's. Women have the ability to experience multiple orgasms since they lack the man's refractory "waiting period" in between ejaculations. Women's orgasms are about 20 seconds longer than a man's on average, and the contractions that take place involve the vagina, uterus and even anus.

Women may also feel a "sex flush," which is a reddening of the skin that happens when blood flow increases. The clitoris becomes erect and the vagina moistens, first in arousal and then in climax. Even physical changes are observed during orgasm, such as the labia minora or inner lips becoming darker in tone, and the clitoris retracting under the hood. The vagina tightens up during orgasm even though it also dilated and expands lengthwise.

One of the things that truly characterizes an orgasm is that it's involuntary. The body "spasms" or "loses control" and experiences all these sensations after an overwhelming assault on all your five senses.

Now here is where sex becomes a slippery slope—pun intended. Even though an orgasm is an involuntary peak and discharge of excitement…

Tip #1: A woman must always want to experience an orgasm. Therefore, she must be made comfortable in the setting and her body and mind must be ready to focus on pleasure.

This is often a misunderstood concept especially when you consider the barrage of BDSM erotica out there. Sure, a woman may enjoy the sensation, the guilt, the taboo of coming against her own will…but *unless she wants it to happen, it's not going to happen.*

A man cannot force a woman to orgasm, no matter if he's Mr. Grey, Dean Winchester,

Don Juan or any other past or present sex symbol. This is because…

Tip #2: An orgasm is as much a mental experience as it is a physical one. A woman must be thoroughly immersed in the erotic experience if an orgasm is to happen.

This means half-assing it, so to speak, or taking ANY negative energy into the sexual experience is a no-no. If a woman's mind is not fully committed to orgasming, all that hand and tongue motion is wasted because she will not allow herself to orgasm.

Besides, even if a man could "force a woman to orgasm" it would probably be a weak level 1 instead of the awe-inspiring level 10 that everyone desires. Yes, believe it or not, not all female orgasms are of the same power, volume or enthusiasm. Just as a man can have a weak "jerk" or a ho-hum ejaculation with hardly any excitement, so too can a woman's orgasm be weak and less than spectacular. So right away we see a major problem—a lack of commitment to making this a truly memorable sexual experience.

Remember, an orgasm is a "discharge of sexual arousal accumulation," so without all that *accumulation* of excitement, from physical and mental stimulation, an orgasm is pretty much empty.

Which takes us to:

Tip #3: Spend more time on the buildup and the arousal stage for a much more intense climax.

So now that we know what an orgasm actually is, and some of the basics of what you're looking for (as an eager to please man or as a woman who wants to teach her man how to get the job done) it's time to go into more depth as to what actually brings about an orgasm. Let's move onto Chapter 2.

Chapter 2: Her Non-Sexual Erogenous Zones

It's actually sort of ridiculous just how recently American men learned how to please women, at least from a purely medical context. Sexually unsatisfied women were once thought to have a condition called "female hysteria" in the 1800s and early 1900s and the cure was a "hysterical paroxysm," which was manual and automatic stimulation of the genitals. It wasn't long before men learned one very simple truth: much like the penis, the vagina had sensitive nerve endings and consistent physical stimulation of these sexual parts was required to induce orgasm—not just the mere act of penetration.

Penetration only activates one "erogenous zone," which is the sensitive nerve endings on the labia minora and the interior entrance of the vaginal wall. However, the entrance of the vulva itself is typically not the most intense of the erogenous zones. Therefore, fast-forwarding to hard pounding, like you typically see in erotica, is not going to do a man any favors when it comes to bringing on orgasm. It may feel good but it's not *enough*.

Instead, learn the erogenous zones point by point and focus on extending foreplay.

Tip #4: Extend pre-penetration foreplay to ensure a woman orgasms at least once—just from foreplay—BEFORE moving onto to penetration.

Not only does this help men ward off premature ejaculation, but it also helps rev up a woman's engine and let her become more aroused—which as we learn, leads to a greater discharge of sexual excitement during orgasm. Even if you make her orgasm from foreplay alone, that's still sexual energy that is "counted" towards an even bigger orgasm building when you start focusing on penetration. There's really no downside to engaging in long minutes or even hours of foreplay—provided she likes what you're doing.

This is where knowing the erogenous zones comes in. There are actually many hot spots on a woman's body that can be properly stimulated, and they start literally at the top of her head and go all the way down to the sole of her feet.

Her Scalp: The scalp and hair follicles of a woman's head are sensitive. No wonder the best kissers always use their hands!

Tip #5: Practice giving her a scalp massage or running fingers through her hair as you kiss or even before.

Mouth: A mouth isn't just for kissing, hollering and sucking you know! The entire mouth, including her lips and tongue are pleasure centers and can be stimulated from sucking, licks and touching.

Tip #6: Spend more time kissing and more time caressing her tongue with your own. Bonus points if you can reach that highly sensitive spot behind and above her upper lip.

Neck: The neck, both the front, side, clavicles (upper shoulder bones), and nape or back of the neck are part of a very sensitive erogenous zone that almost always precedes moving to "second base."

Tip #7: Once you know that a woman is highly sensitive when you touch or kiss her neck, don't try to rush things forward. Instead, dwell on it longer. If she's excited enough to let a man touch her breasts or genitals, just from kissing…imagine the response you could get by lip and hand caressing all crevices of the neck. You could even gently bite her and leave a love hickey, which some women really respond to.

Ears: Ears are very sensitive spots and all the more so on and behind the earlobe. Don't underestimate the power of an erotic whisper.

Tip #8: Whisper sexy things in her ear, or breathe softly into her ear. Then, lick, caress, kiss or gently bite her earlobe or the area behind it. It's hard not to feel excited when this happens, since ears are so closely connected to aural input, which is so connected to emotion!

Breasts: The nipple and surrounded areola area have many nerve endings, and so much concentration that some women can actually orgasm just with breast play. Theories on why they are more sensitive than other spots include (A) tiny hair follicles surrounding areola; (B) smooth muscle and glandular-duct tissue prevents development of the usual dermal nerve networks, present in less explosive erogenous zones; production of oxytocin and prolactin, after stimulation, which affects the genitals.

Tip #9: Increase breast foreplay and spend more time kissing, sucking, gently biting, caressing and squeezing the nipples and areola.

Tip #10: Don't forget to play with the breast tissue and skin itself, giving attention to all parts of her body.

Tease her by starting with breast tissue touching then making her wait for direct nipple stimulation. Start slow and soft, with touches or caresses and progress into tighter squeezing.

Stomach: The stomach, the abdomen and naval, are all highly sensitive areas since they are close to the pubic bone. It's no coincidence that dress fashions have always hidden the belly, while ancient Taoism has glorified the belly and pubic region as part of the complete "yoni" area, the essence of the feminism spirit.

Some speculation states that the navel and genitals of a women may actually have the same type of tissue, hence the most intense reactions to touch.

Tip #11: Spend more time licking, touching and caressing a woman's belly. Before going anywhere near the genitals, treat her belly as a forbidden part, and penetrate her naval with your tongue or finger. Some women report feeling a direct jolt of excitement that travels up their spine when their naval is aroused.

Tailbone: It's actually far more likely that your average woman is going to find tailbone stimulation more arousing than direct anal sex. As we will discuss below, the anal cavity has no actual nerve endings except indirect stimulation of vaginal spots; therefore, the only direct nerve stimulation south of the vagina would be indirect touching around the tailbone area.

Tip #12: Caress, kiss or stimulate the tailbone which is located right above the anus near the base of her spine and right below where the top of the butt cheeks divide. The middle

finger may be able to reach this area "hooking" on in a natural shape.

Arms: Some women have admitted that elbow caressing can actually bring them to orgasm in some cases. This is because the softer skin of the inner side of the arms, especially around the mid-arm bend, is an erogenous zone.

Tip #13: Use your fingers or tongue to caress a woman's inner elbow, starting slow and then increasing pressure just as if you were playing with the genitals. While it's not sure to bring on orgasm it can oftentimes start clitoral or vaginal arousal.

Finger: Fingertips have nerve endings and are highly sensitive to light touching. They are actually considered the second-most sensitive part after the tongue.

Tip #14: Practice touching your partner for fun and experiment with different caresses, licks, kisses and touches. Travel from the fingertips to the palm, back hand and even the web of skin between fingers.

Legs: Thighs are very sensitive areas, as are the back of the legs and the bending point and the front knees.

Tips #15: Use your caressing hands or lips or tongue to explore this erogenous zone.

Kissing a woman's thighs for at least a few moments, and eventually working your way to the labia majora, and then minora, (outer and inner lips) almost always precedes direct genital stimulation. Moving too fast to the clitoris may be too intense and cause discomfort. Make sure she's wet by stimulating the thighs and outer lips until you feel her wetness.

Feet: Feet worshiping is not necessarily a fetish, considering how many nerve endings there are in the sole of a foot as well as the toes. Some even theorize that feet stimulation is similar in brain function to genital stimulation. This could explain why some women can get turned on by sucking toes, licking feet, or even kissing the top of her foot.

Tips #16: Try kissing and caressing her feet and working your way up from the feet to the ankles, legs, and eventually thighs giving a full body massage and sensual caress.

Other Parts: Of course there are plenty of other spots on a woman's body that may be neglected—and rather than assuming that only erogenous zones deserve attention, you can try experimenting with touches, massages, caresses and licking or stroking. Some women really enjoy having their shoulders rubbed, or their back. Sometimes fetishes like armpit licking or even anal sex can be a turn on, but it's not the sort of thing you take as a definite thing. This is why you …

Tips #17: Communicate beforehand and during sexual foreplay.

You can discuss what she likes done or you can simply do it and notice how she responds. For instance, if she starts breathing faster or moaning after rubbing her shoulders or kissing the back of her neck, then that's a positive sign that you can keep doing the same. Silence or too much laughter obviously means it's not working and it's time to move on. It's just a matter of listening to a woman's body.

Tip #18: Learn to love a woman's body.

The less goal-oriented you are, the better lover you're going to become. Take your time and explore her body, avoiding her genitals altogether, until you've really taken the time to learn her every curve.

In Tantric sex and "sensate focus," a type of sexual therapy influenced by Tantra, for example, lovers are instructed to not try to make each other orgasm and to avoid touching the genitals, since this creates the pressure to have sex, orgasm and be done with it in record time. Instead, your intent should be removing the goal of orgasm altogether so that you can learn what a woman actually DOES find stimulating and the sensations she does want to experience.

No pressure to orgasm means no worrying about orgasmic response. It will force the two of you to get creative and have fun with each other's non sexual body parts and simply live the sensations you create—the subtle variations in touch, in emotion and in gradual buildup of sexual anticipation.

If a man takes his time and learns to love a woman's body, eventually she's going to beg him to give her the good stuff. If you've done foreplay right, you're at a great place and are ready to bring it up a notch and include genital stimulation.

Now we're getting into the meat of the situation, er, pun intended. Yes, it is reasonable to think that all foreplay eventually ends with direct vaginal and or clitoral stimulation. The fact is that not all women will be capable of orgasming from foreplay and even if they do, they may still crave a stronger clitoral and vaginal orgasm—and yes, some women admit that there is a different in intensity.

Understanding the anatomy of the vagina is a must, as well as various nerve concentrations inside. This is what we'll be discussing Chapter 3.

Chapter 3: Inside the Vagina

The most common mistakes men make in bed is that they either:

- Obsess over doing just one maneuver until the woman comes (and she often doesn't and so he runs out of ideas)

- Don't remain flexible or curious but are too focused on achieving a goal

- Don't understand anatomy

- Don't understand how specifically to stimulate each part of a woman's genitals

This is why

Tips #19 is: give attention to her entire vagina over the course of your foreplay well before finishing with penetration.

The more you play with her genitals in advance of penetration, the moister she will be and the easier it will be for her to come from penetration—especially if she's already orgasmed from foreplay.

Just as we learned to take non-genital foreplay slow in the previous chapter—so much that you avoid touching the vagina altogether at first—it's time to SLOWLY learn the vaginal anatomy and give equal attention to all parts.

Even though internet education and even comedy TV shows has actually taught men a great deal about the clitoris' existence in recent years, a lot of men still don't quite understand that the clitoris is DIRECTLY related to a woman's total orgasmic experience. Sigmund Freud once taught that a clitoral orgasm was immature and a vaginal orgasm belonged to a more mature woman. While he may have been vaguely onto something (as we'll discuss more about G-spot orgasms later) he still failed to see that the clitoris operates as the sort of center-chamber of a woman's body. Even if you achieve a G-spot or A-spot orgasm, it all encompasses nerve endings that stretch back to the clitoris.

In fact, studies show that the vagina itself, apart from the entrance walls and inner lips, is not as sensitive as the clitoris itself. The lower third (closer to the entrance) has the most nerve endings, and the most nerve endings means the most orgasmic potential.

In contrast the two inner thirds of the vagina canal are not as sensitive, and this is also the part that most men think they want to "pound", "obliterate" and "fuck hard" according to the porn vocabulary. According to what we know about nerve endings however, that may be wasted energy.

Now that's not to say that exploring inner vagina is a waste of time, no, you should explore it along with clitoral stimulation. But instead of just pounding away…

Tip #20: Learn where each intervaginal erogenous zone is located.

This means:

- The Clitoris
- The G-Spot
- The A-Spot
- The U-Spot
- The P-Spot

This is probably more spots than you anticipated! But the good news is that most of these areas can be stimulated by your tongue, finger, penis or even a long toy.

Just to clarify:

The G-Spot

The Grafenberg Spot refers to a patch of ribbed and tougher part of vaginal tissue that is located on the anterior (front wall of the vagina) about two to three inches inside. It is sometimes compared to the roof of a woman's mouth (the sensitive behind-the-lip palate we discussed earlier) and feels sponge-like when a woman becomes closer to orgasm. This is usually the spot linked with female squirting or ejaculation, discussed later.

Not everyone actually believes in the G-spot's unique existence; though there are clearly nerve endings there, some believe it is merely an extension of the clitoris.

The A-Spot

The A-spot refers to the anterior fornix, which is located on the same anterior wall that holds the G-spot but is about two to three inches farther inside. The AFE spot is actually near the cervix, which is actually "too far in" for most women and will cause pain. The trick would be to find the A-spot right before you find the cervix. Like the G-spot, the A-spot is also associated with female squirting since it's often called a degenerated prostate, and also is suggested to activate a woman's bladder. A-spot stimulation is actually recommended for vaginal dryness since it does sometimes stimulate a woman's wetness.

The U Spot

The U-spot is not frequently mentioned even in sex education and is a somewhat fetishistic idea that is just now becoming more mainstream. This refers not to the urethra itself but the tissue just above it, the area right in between the clitoris and urethra, which is for urinating. However, the pleasurable feelings associated with the spot can sometimes reach as far as the urethral opening in addition to the tissue. Stroking, licking or tapping this area can sometimes increase arousal giving a new sort of U-spot mini-orgasm.

The P Spot and Deep Spot

These two spots are perhaps the most controversial erogenous zones, as they arguably are the only anal stimulation—besides the tail bone area previously discussed—that's scientifically based. The P-Spot is the posterior fornix and is opposite the A-spot, but passed the cervix. Supposedly it can only be reached using fingers, certain positions or toys.

Meanwhile, the Deep Spot, or Rectouterine Pouch, also called the Cul-De, Sac is the patch of skin found in between the rectum and the posterior. The only way to reach it would be deep vaginal penetration or perhaps anal intercourse, for a more indirect feeling. This could explain why some women have anal orgasms, though the consensus at this time seems to be that anal orgasms are only mentally induced. Another way to reach the deep spot is with a middle finger, but turned downward, reverse of the G-spot come hither movement. By pushing downward, you may actually activate the deep spot and trigger what feels like an anal orgasm from deep vaginal pressing.

And here in lies the dilemma for so many men. They understand the anatomy, or at least are capable of learning where each "part" is.

But they don't actually learn how to stimulate a woman's body or these pressure points adequately.

The result is stressful, embarrassing and downright unsexy. Trying to make her feel something when you don't actually know how to do it right. So in the coming chapter, pun intended(!) we're going to actually discuss techniques that will help you to locate and pinpoint these spots for greater arousal and orgasmic release. Let's start with the most basic: the clitoris.

Chapter 4: The Clitoris—How Find the Hot Spot

The clitoris is simply the most "erogenously-inclined" part of a woman's vagina and is located near the front of the labia minora or inner lips. It is above the urethra, which is used for urination. It is the most sensitive part of a woman's body and the only part used solely for sexual stimulation.

Interestingly, in nature, what starts as a "genital tubercle" will grow into either a penis or clitoris, depending on the gender of the person. So the clitoris is the female equivalent of a penis, and it's simply illogical not to include clitoral orgasms as part of your foreplay—and even incidentally part of penetration.

The clitoris is about the size of a pea and is believed to have a whopping 8,000 nerve endings. Of course you know by now that a clitoris can be:

- Fingered
- Licked
- Kissed
- Sucked
- Or manipulated by a dildo or vibrator

However, we're going to leave the choice of how the lady likes it up to you. Instead, let's focus on the physical motions that allow for clitoral stimulation.

Fingering Techniques

Tip #21: Always trim your nails and make sure they are not sharp if you're going to use your fingers. If you're using your tongue, start slow and make sure she's comfortable and then work your way up to a faster rhythm.

Tip #22: The up and down maneuver should be used on ONE SIDE of the clitoris.

Remember that direct contact is very intense and may be too much at the beginning, so start with a side touch and then if necessary you can do direct contact with an up and down motion.

Tip #23: The round-up maneuver sees you using all four fingers in a circular motion, touching both the CLITORIS AND LABIA. Not as much direct clitoris pressure but better when starting.

Tip #24: The side-to-side maneuver sees you running one or two fingers side to side directly over the clitoris. However, varying your fingers, the pressure and combination maneuvers with up and down and side to side works best, so experimentation is key.

Tip #25: Squeezing the clitoris is an often neglected move that can stimulate a woman's arousal and all you have to do is put your thumb and index finger on both sides and then press downward and inward, with GENTLE squeezes.

The clitoris is not as sensitive as, say, a man's balls—so you can apply a little more pressure if she's comfortable. ROLL IT

AROUND after squeezing for an additional effect.

Tip #26: Tap the clitoris with your fingertips. Not everyone will find this arousing but some will. Make sure the clitoris is exposed by pulling the lips back and out of the way and then tap your finger tip gently on the clit head.

The clitoris should not be thought of as a button, nor as a penis. While you do jerk it up and down slightly, like a penis, it is not as instantly responsive as a man's penis. Fast-forwarding to a full-on clit massage may be too intense for comfort, and that's not always a good thing.

Therefore, easing into it is pivotal. And this means not only starting slow but…

Tip #27: Paying attention to areas AROUND the clitoris. Stimulating these areas will warm her up and make her more responsive to firmer movements.

Therefore parts like:

- The clitoral hood

- The clitoral shaft

- The labia minora lips
- The labia majora
- The urethra and surrounding tissue

Tip #29: Stimulate her inner shaft of the clitoris by pushing down on the woman's lower abdomen with your fingers. Massage the skin on one side of her vagina as if making scissors. This will make the surrounding inner labia naturally caress her shaft.

Tip #30: Spend more time with the clitoral hood and inner lips, rubbing them in the same way as an up and down clit massaging motion.

Tip #31: Put your hand on her pubic bone, using your palm to push back the upper skin on her lower abdomen, while your spread fingers rest on her pubic hair.

Tip #32: You can also push her labia lips, clitoral hood upwards, when ready, to get more direct clitoral stimulation—usually after she's been aroused from incidental touching.

The only thing left to say is be responsive and react according to how she feels. Need a clue? You don't only have to rely on sighs and moans. Look for physical changes in the clit and surrounding tissue areas like:

Tip #33: The clitoris hides then becomes aroused and exposed, then hides again when she is on the brink of orgasm.

The clit tip is pulled back under the hood when she's ready to orgasm, so pressing the lips upward and getting a better direct touch may be necessary. You can also tell if she's ready to orgasm if contractions are starting inside her vagina or around the pubic mound.

While there is a whole section devoted to masturbation later on, for now, know that these fingering exercises apply whether you're a lover pleasuring a woman or are a woman learning to touch yourself for the first time.

But what happens when touching isn't enough? Then it's time to break out your secret weapon...The Tongue.

Oral Sex Techniques

Kissing, licking and tongue flicking the clitoris is just as effective, if not more effective, since the tongue is naturally soft, firm and self-lubricating, as opposed to fingers which can be dry and sometimes irritating to sensitive skin.'

However, just as fingers can be misused, tongues can also be downright lizardly and creepy if not used strategically! So remember what we already learned—taking it slow. Start by stimulating the outer and inner labia with your lips, and then her lower abdomen and pubic mound BEFORE arriving at her clit.

Tip #34: Once you arrive at the clitoris take it slow by choosing a RHYTHM that you can consistently do for several minutes without wearing yourself out.

For some, it helps to think of you signing your name with your tongue or perhaps licking each letter of the alphabet in cursive. This allows your tongue to build a rhythm while also going in various directions and speeds. If you sense or hear that one letter really drives her crazy REPEAT it.

Tip #35: Suck and lick at the same time.

When she is aroused, and the clit becomes engorged with blood, grab it between your LIPS and hold it. Suck it while you lick or flick it with your tongue. As she gets more excited increase your tongue speed and the power of your suction.

Tip #36: Some people have the ability to roll their tongue and if you can do it, that means you can tongue roll around a woman's clit and give a side winding tongue massage.

Place the clit between both sides of your rolled tongue and then move it back and forth in the middle. It's almost the equivalent of "deep throating a clitoris"; just make sure she's properly excited and her clitoris is popping out before attempting.

Tip #37: Hum your way to a symphony by actually humming with your mouth while you lick and suck her clitoris.

When the clit is stimulated with extra vibration is adds to the intensity. However, you don't need a vibrator since you can make these vibrations with your voice. Hum softly using your soft lips directly on her clitoris and then as she gets excited hum just a little harder and louder.

Naturally, the clitoris is a flexible organ and so the less you limit yourself in technique the better. You don't even have to stop at fingering or oral sex. Certain sexual positions and penis maneuvers can help achieve orgasm. For instance...

Tip #38: Use a sexual position to cause friction on this clitoris.

The easiest way to do this is to simply rub your erect penis on the woman's clit. However, you can also cause additional stimulation by:

- Missionary position (she bends her knees slightly)

- Thigh grinding (She sits almost reverse cow girl but clasps her legs around his thigh, putting her clit against his thigh and then grinding on him)

- Kneeling missionary (Both lovers kneel on a bed in front of each other, facing each other, and with their genitals lined up and the man's erection pushing into her clit)

- Doggy style (From this position a man can use his penis penetrating from behind or reach around with his hands to rub the clitoris)

Tip #39: Whatever you do, don't stop.

Much like a rough blowjob causes a man's penis as much intense feeling as it does pleasure, a throbbing clit during orgasm is usually helped by CONTINUING stimulation—even if it seems like her body is telling you to stop. The only way she'll want you to stop is if it hurts, which is typically will not. However, it will be intense and while she is contracting she wants you to keep the same motion going—not stopping and starting a new rhythm but keeping the same pace as is. Do not stop just because a woman is already screaming and spasming. Once she relaxes, the clitoris becomes sensitive again and she may need her own "waiting period", meaning just a few minutes or seconds to start up again. It's not as long as a refractory period so as soon as she's ready to try again, indulge her.

Remember that a woman's blood flows freely through her tissues after she reaches the point of orgasm, and this makes multiples easier.

The clitoris loves experimentation, but that experimenting should always be balanced with consistent RHYTHM, just like a song has its own recurring pattern. Like Stairway to Heaven…always popular with the ladies. Find a technique that works and keep it going until you're just about ready to die! This is why it's strongly recommended to start at a slower pace, one that you're comfortable with doing for a long while, and not start out so roughly that you wear you and her out.

As if the clitoris isn't complex enough, now it's time to meet the even more elusive and "unexplained" G-Spot. This is the focus of our next chapter.

Chapter 5: The G-Spot—Myths and Facts about the Big Squirt

The G-Spot is controversial to say the least, since there are women who claim not to have them, and even sexologists and researchers who claim they don't technically exist. Their explanations usually consist of:

- They are complete myths and all mental climax

- They are part of the tail end of the clitoris

- There are nerve endings there, but there is no such thing as female "squirt" (it's just pee)

Of course, some sexologists do believe in the G-spot and more importantly, there are millions of anecdotes coming from women who claimed to have experienced them. So first things first:

Tip #40: A woman shouldn't feel obligated to have a G-spot orgasm.

Look for it, experiment, and see if she feels anything. Don't fret about it if it doesn't happen because there are plenty more hot spots to look for.

As stated earlier, the G-spot is a hypothetical center of nerve endings seemingly separate from the clitoris, but one that is still connected at some level. Sigmund Freud's belief that vaginal orgasms were "mature" was not terribly far off from the truth. Stimulating the G-spot is a "different" orgasm than just a clitoral orgasm. Most women say that it feels more whole body, and may also allow them multiple orgasms, whereas clitoral orgasms require a bit of a waiting period because of the sensitivity of the clitoris.

Most controversially, it lets women ejaculate or "squirt", though research is divided on whether this is pee, some special female equivalent of prostate fluid found in the paraurethral gland, or even old urine that has been altered with other elements. Regardless of what it is…

Tip #41: Help a woman feel relaxed about a G-spot orgasm and "squirting" letting her know there's nothing to be embarrassed about and you want to experience it with her.

Tip #42: Start by tongue penetrating her, not only with the clitoris but into her vagina, tasting her fluid.

This will help her come, especially if you stick to the outer area where most nerve endings are. The more she orgasms previously, the more susceptible she will be to a G-spot orgasm.

Understand the shape and feel of the area. It's about the size of a quarter and is bean-shaped. You can differentiate it from the rest of her vaginal canal but identifying rougher patches of skin, about 1-3 inches back from the front vaginal entrance. It is on the same side as her belly. The G-spot is nothing but a series of erectile tissues which explains why a woman has to be pre-aroused so that blood can rush into the area.

Tip #43: Find it by inserting two fingers and making the come hither gesture.

Adding lubricant always seems to help as a dry vagina will not make the already elusive spot any easier to find.

Tip #44: Gauge her reaction.

Feeling the desire to pee is usually a telling sign that you're activating it and it's not actual pee, just a passing feeling. (Of course, for the purpose of making her feel comfortable you have to let her know that you're okay with urine and you're not going to freak out! Women can be very self-conscious about this)

Tip #45: You may have to vary the manner in which you stimulate the G-spot.

If she feels nothing then vary the speed, perhaps doing it faster than slower. Or changing from light pressure to heavier pressure. You can also vary the light flicking movements to more intense RUBBING, or CIRCULAR, or SCOOPING OUT or SIDE TO SIDE. Much like the clitoris, different motions may lead to different reactions.

Tip #46: Use your other hand on the mons pubis area, right above the pubic bone and where hair grows, and massage it gently.

This sometimes helps intensify the feeling. Sitting on her stomach may also be a prime position, since this automatically provides the additional front wall pressure.

Tip #47: When all else fails, add clitoral stimulation.

It certainly can't hurt and even if the G-spot doesn't happen all the extra caressing will still intensify the clitoral orgasm. Stimulate the clitoris and G-spot together—this is where most women report female ejaculation.

Tip #48: Move your G-spot positioning slightly if there is no reaction or if she feels the urge to urinate too strongly.

Much like the clitoris is overly sensitive, so too can the G-spot be too intense to stimulate directly. In this case, move your fingers over slightly, going to the 11 and 1 o'clock position, with two fingers, rather than the traditional 12 spot.

Tip #49: Use sexual positions that heighten G-spot friction.

These include:

- A woman lying on her back with a pillow elevating her butt.

- Doggy style with hand stimulation from behind

- A woman on top, since she has more room to move around and find the G-spot herself.

- Legs over shoulders. She can easily lift her pelvis off the bed (or use pillows) so that deeper penetration and G-spot grazing is possible. If you align correctly, the angle of her hips allows for his penis to rub almost directly against the front vaginal wall, firmly pressing the G-spot with every thrust.

Tip #50: Get your partner to help you.

A woman can help herself G-spot orgasm by pressing down on her lower abdomen while her partner continues with G-spot or clitoris stimulation. In addition, some women claim that if they do a mini-crunch on their abdominal muscles, like a half-sit up could help.

Tip #51: Try to stuff more than one finger inside when looking for the G-spot and go in farther than you need to, just so your knuckles can massage her internally back and forth, side by side.

If a women is determined to have one (and obviously if she's close-minded to it, it probably won't happen) then strengthening pelvic muscles (PC) muscle contractions can help. This is the flex she can do to stop the flow of urination.

Last but not least, don't give up. According to some research, women peak sexually at 30 and after and sometimes find G-spot orgasms easier to achieve than in their 20s. This is believed to have something to do with the hormone estrogen, which may make the vaginal wall too thick to find the G-spot. Since the 30s minimizes this hormone, the wall and G-spot may actually become easier to find with age.

All you can really know for sure is that an open-mind—yours and hers—is the most effective way to produce an outstanding, out of this world orgasm. Always make sure you're comfortable above all else and aren't putting any emotional pressure on her to come vigorously. Sometimes exploring is really the best part of the process.

Speaking of which, it's about time we explored something completely new to the old G-spot and clitoris argument. What about the latest cutting edge research that suggests there are multiple spots within the vagina, beside the big two, that can improve orgasmic response? Let's review how to find them in Chapter 6.

Chapter 6: The U-Spot, A-Spot, P-Spot and Deep Spot

What about all those other mysterious spots that many man have sought to explore and conquer, but few have actually found? There is good evidence to suggest that there are other centers of nerve endings in the vagina and it all really depends on how far you want to go—literally speaking, as the deeper you go, the more spots you find.

The U-Spot

The U-spot, as stated earlier, is merely the urethra and surrounding tissue area from where she pees. This is located right above her vagina but below the clitoris. Stimulation of the urethra is not comparable to the G-spot or clit, which do require some significant power. It's actually better to very lightly touch or tickle the opening of the urethra. Speaking of female squirting, in theory this is where ejaculate comes out of, even if it's not urine. So there's certainly nothing to lose, and yet a lot to gain, by…

Tip #52: Pay some attention to the U-spot, at least when also caressing the clitoral hood, lips and clitoris.

Tickle the urethra surroundings and then very lightly the hole itself when working in other massages, like the clit and vagina. Focusing too much individual attention on the urethra might make a woman uncomfortable.

The A-Spot

The A-spot we already revealed as a spot one stop further than the G-spot and along the same front wall. Much like the G-spot, proper positioning (usually lying on her back) is important, as is lubricant.

Tip #53: Stick a finger inside and try to reach the deepest point.

You will feel an area that is spongy, like the G-spot. However, the cervix is actually near the A-spot, and this feels a bit different—rounder, firmer and a bit like rubber. Practically all women will find the cervix uncomfortable so listen to her, and be careful about pushing in too far.

One misconception is that the A-spot is far back into the vagina and inaccessible for most men. Not true at all, it's just a matter of not understanding the position. The G-spot is not far in at all, and may be as short a distance from the entrance as 1-2 inches. Therefore, 3-4 inches is all you need to reach the A-spot with a finger or penis. The vaginal canal itself is, on average, less than four inches long, from the entrance to the cervix.

The intent is to start rubbing the area, just as with the G-spot until she starts lubricating. The creation of pressure and rhythm that characterizes clit stimulation, and even penetration, also serves the purpose here. Apply a scooping motion if simple stroking doesn't seem to work. Some experts believe that practicing stimulating the area on a regular basis, like 10 minutes a day, may help to make lubrication and orgasm easier.

The P-Spot and Deep Spot

It's best to combine these two spots because not only are they often confused with each other, as well as the A-spot (which is actually NOT as "deep" a spot) but in practical terms you are going to come so close to both of them that you (the man) or she is likely not going to notice the subtle differences between the posterior fornix and the rectouterine pouch or cul-de-sac. The only real difference in location is that the P-spot is past the A-spot on the front wall and rectouterine pouch is on the bottom wall, accessible only with deep thrusting or maybe anal sex.

Frankly, both of these spots are going to be difficult unless the man is particularly well endowed, but even if so, it's simply more anatomically correct to use a long dildo or even your fingers to find the spot, at least when you first start looking for it. A twisting motion as your fingers are deep inside her might do the trick, and especially if you stimulate her G-spot or A-spot and clitoris at the same time using your index finger, middle finger and thumb for the clit.

Tip #54: Once you know where the area is, use a sexual position for more natural stimulation.

In terms of fingering, have her lay in rear-entry or doggy style position and then using a toy or finger might work, as this will give you greater access and more focused concentration. However, some women can have their deep spot stimulated with just rear-entry penetration. The Deep Missionary Position can also help, as the penis tip reaches the anterior fornix or A-spot.

The fornices (plural) might as well be one erogenous zone, but just know that if you were to actually reach the P-spot it would be very close to the cervix. This explains why many women both love and hate the idea of deep penetration. Because one wrong move, one inch too far and you're hitting the cervix. The cervix actually requires stimulation to move out of the way and allow a deeper thrust into the fornices, but this is not easy.

So don't be surprised if women do not like deep thrusting that pounds against the cervix; some women who use long and straight dildos says finding the A-spot is uncomfortable enough but going hard for the deep spot / P-spot is downright scary if you don't know what you're doing. Remember a sharp jab into the cervix may even kill her mood entirely so if you're going to tread in dangerous territory go SLOW and ask for feedback.

Not to demotivate you to try—after all, some women say that if you find the deep spot and can penetrate, it feels more long-lasting as if coming from a deeper part of the woman's abdomen.

Tip #55: Definitely plan to use lubricant with a dildo or finger, as this eases the friction which is public enemy number one when it comes to deep vaginal penetration.

And yes this tip bears repeating…

Tip #56: Do NOT be satisfied with penetration or intercourse alone.

It always works best in COMBINATION. Clitoral, G-spot, A-spot, deep spot, P-spot and U-spot simulation, it's all good. The more you touch her and explore her body, never losing track of her #1 Erogenous Zone, the clit, the better.

Up until now, we've been discussing plenty of anatomy and the best way to stimulate the erogenous zones—as opposed to mindless thrusting that does nothing special. However, the next few chapters are going to focus on something even more important than "her hot spots", her "buttons" and "the motion of the ocean."

Her mental and emotional connection to her lover. If she doesn't feel this then anatomy won't matter much. Let's start by discussing the most common cause and solution of anorgasmia (the inability to orgasm) — mental resistance to physical pleasure.

Chapter 7: The Elusive Mental Orgasm

Orgasm is all about mental and emotional connection and the excitement that comes from that connection. Believe it or not, even a man as ready to orgasm as he is, will find emotional and mentally "fueled" orgasms much more intense than just a hot rough quickie.

In fact, mental orgasms if you can train yourself to have them, as a man or a woman, are going to be your best friend all the way into your 60s and 70s, even if your genitals slow down. Because mental orgasms are powerful and can give you the same euphoric feelings as ejaculation.

Whereas this an optional process for men, it's really a must for a woman. That's not to say that mental orgasm is all about "love" or romance. No, it's about immersion in the experience itself, the emotional connection with another human being.

The fact is that the most recent scientific evidence suggests that orgasm itself IS a mental process that triggers a physical process, not the other way around. Actually, many people claim to be able to think their way to orgasm regardless of organ touching, penetration or any friction whatsoever. The theory is that it's all a matter of brain chemistry, since the pleasure centers of the brain that show activity in a woman "thinking herself to orgasm" show practically the same level of activity for a woman who reaches orgasm by physical stimulation. And these brain centers that show said activity, do not do the same thing when a woman "fakes" it. Research concluded that orgasm is a mental process and one very unique to each women since it takes a variety of emotional triggers to help her reach this state.

What about physical friction? Isn't it necessary in some degree, since physical factors (including a romantic and sexy environment) can help a woman to feel pleasure and comfort? Yes, but the physical factors are stimuli she is taking in to help her begin the mental orgasmic process. She consciously chooses to allow her orgasm to start, and continue, as her body begins helping her mind achieve arousal.

In addition, when a woman comes, the physical "symptoms" of orgasm happen the same way no matter WHAT activity brings it on the process of:

- Erogenous Zone stimulation
- Increase in heart rate, blood pressure and breathing
- Tension inside the pelvis
- Contracting muscles in all areas of the pelvis
- Release of tension and afterglow

All of this happens, even if a woman THINKS herself to orgasm, the mental process triggers physical actions. Even people with spinal cord injuries, as studies have told us (Sipski et al. 2006) have reported being able to reach orgasm, despite not having proper use of their genitals.

So we get it—orgasm is mental, but how does this relate to giving a woman a powerful, mind-blowing orgasm? Simply because, if she has subconscious resistance to orgasming, she will not orgasm. She will not pull those "triggers" and allow her mind to come, and this will block her ability to physically come—no matter if you thrust for hours.

Now that said, if you do apply pressure to an erogenous zone, she will feel pleasure. Just as touching your penis provides pleasure, so does touching those spots that we discussed in the female anatomy. However, orgasm is about LOSING CONTROL and letting go of inhibitions. This is why it's very difficult if not impossible to force a woman to orgasm if she's feeling disconnected from the experience.

The most common reasons for this disconnect are:

- Anxiety or self-doubt

- Lack of trust

- Performance anxiety or undue pressure to orgasm

- Fear or ignorance of sex, orgasm and erogenous zones

- Fear of losing control

- Relationship problems

So the first thing you as a conscientious lover need to do is…

Tip #57: Make sure she is trusting, ready to enjoy herself and there is no subconscious resistance to you helping her come.

That's right—HELPING her come. You are not MAKING her come.

A woman must first decide she's comfortable enough to orgasm. This doesn't necessarily mean romantic feelings or even feelings of trust. But she must be confident enough in the environment to perform, surrender to her lover, and allow the mental process of orgasm to begin.

Part of this obligation you have is to:

Tip #58: Create a comfortable environment. One that does not scare her, make her uncomfortable or fill her head with unsexy thoughts.

Tip #59: Assure her, or show her, that she can do no wrong. That you are completely happy and ready to see her orgasm, on her own terms, with no special requests.

If she does not feel this self-confidence, she will quickly develop performance anxiety and will not feel comfortable orgasming. She may even want to…but she will not be able to.

It is your job to make sure that your lover is:

- Secure in her body
- Confident in her sexy personality
- Secure about how she tastes, smells and feels
- Secure in her voice, personality and her unique self-view
- Excited to orgasm and fully confident that you won't laugh, or be embarrassed, or act "weird" about anything she's about to do.

You can reassure her by your words and your actions.

Tip #60: Tell her she is good in everything, from taste to smell to behavior.

Everyone's a little self-conscious about their "O-Face" but you must put all these fears to rest. Tell her she's sexy and put some emotion into it, deepening your voice, making strong eye contact, and being confident yourself.

Tip #61: Give her the same reassurances physically.

Touch her often, and always give her the impression that you're having fun and that you're not feeling frustrated or impatient. Make noise, showing your sexual arousal, and get in touch with your caveman instincts, touching and caressing her body, letting her know YOU DESIRE HER.

Sex is definitely not the time to make her feel insecure or play mind games. This is the arena where she needs to hear your support.

This all seems logical, right? A woman has full power over her body and won't give you the gift of her orgasm unless she feels it naturally. However, there is another major issue to consider and it's one of the most common factors cited in women who cannot seem to "do it right."

A lack of education and experience. Let's talk about getting in touch with yourself…no literally! Touching yourself.

Chapter 8: Masturbation — Back to School, Folks!

This is a surprisingly common scenario—a woman sits back and lies there, wondering why she can't orgasm. Maybe something's wrong with her. Maybe she's one of those women who just can't orgasm for some strange and obscure medical reason.

No, while there is such a thing as anorgasmia (discussed later) the truth is most women who sit back and lie there waiting to orgasm have been given MISINFORMATION about sex or are completely ignorant as to their own bodies.

This happens more commonly than you might think, and it's not just among conservative society who do not engage in premarital sex for experience. Even among the worldly wise and sexually active, many girls are deceived into thinking that it's the man's obligation to "give her an orgasm," when it's actually HER job to do it, and to either (A) let the man help her using his own strategies, or (B) show the man how she wants it done.

Of course, women who have no sex education to fall back on, watch movies, or read erotic, or see porn, which warps and exaggerates the entire sexual encounter, showing that women just come on demand, because a man is JUST that dominant. Yeah, right.

The woman holds all the cards here, folks. And if she has no idea how to orgasm ON HER OWN, then she has no idea how to orgasm with a partner. It's going to be awkward, disappointing and maybe even traumatizing.

This is why:

Tip #62: A woman should be able to masturbate and bring herself to orgasm.

So help her orgasm. Or if necessary, let her orgasm on her own while you lay there and watch. She has to do this for herself—it's part of the sexually maturing process.

First, she has to be comfortable coming in your presence. If she's not confident to do just that, this is indicative of a bigger relationship or communication problem. She has to be happy and excited enough to come and give you the pleasure of watching her.

Next, she has to be knowledgeable of what she's touching, where, why and how.

It's astonishing that a lot of women have never actually looked at their vagina in the mirror and masturbated. Maybe they feel this is a dirty thing to do, or a silly thing to do, since sex is going to be "Oh So Easy" to figure out. Wrong! Why waste time masturbating if you can find someone to have sex with? Wrong again.

This is not a dirty thing or a silly thing but a LEARNING PROCESS. If you (man or woman) don't learn what you have down there, you're not going to understand:

- How to use it

- How you like to be touched

- How much intensity is too much as to be painful

- How much intensity is too much to control (premature orgasm)

- How you can use your body to please someone else

- Where your erogenous zones are

- What unique rhythms (touching, pressure, speed, strength) you enjoy

This is sex 101 and if you skip this unique lesson in learning yourself you're always going to have a hard time orgasming "on demand" the way we would all like. Or, if you're a man, you're never going to be able to get a predictable orgasm, because it will be a big mystery that neither you understand nor she understands.

Steps of Learning the Female Orgasm (for Women)

The first step is orgasming alone and in one's own presence.

The second step is looking to see what is happening (a mirror is best recommended) and how it feels.

The third step is to either let a partner experiment with your body to feel new sensations or guide him to do what you know is going to feel good.

With some experience in female anatomy, a man may be able to guide a woman to an orgasm just by knowing what works for most. But, over time, the man will discover that each woman has a unique formula that brings her to orgasm, a combination of physical movements, mental thoughts and volatile emotions. This is why masturbating on one's own, and then in the presence of a lover, is important:

- For the woman to learn herself.

- For the man to learn the woman and what she needs to get over the edge.

Masturbation Techniques

This section is written from the female point of view, though you as a man may have to explain it to an inexperienced woman at some point.

The Water Fall: Understandably, a lot of women are shy when it comes to touching themselves for the first time, and so using a bathroom faucet or shower head may be the best way to start the self-pleasuring process.

Tip #63: Let a medium to strong stream of water land on your clitoris.

Sit at the end of the tub, sliding your butt down, with low water and position yourself so that it will fall on the clitoris. Avoid getting too much water directly into the vagina since this can cause physical problems. Make sure the pressure is light (perhaps starting with one finger over the faucet, creating a small sprinkle) and the water is warm, not hot. Progress to more rapid streams as you go along.

You can also get an extra potent jolt from a Jacuzzi tub with its jet streams that can land on your clitoris creating intensity even from a distance.

The Vibrator: The vibrator is your second best friend in life, as it really is made to perform every action you or a man could, by providing slow-to-fast pulsations on any erogenous zone you want. While vibrators are typically used for clit stimulation, there are also products for G-spot stimulation (with curved shafts, for reaching the anterior wall), anal or vaginal "bead" stimulator (which are pulled out) and advanced vibrators that actually offer multiple motions, speeds and thrusting styles at once.

Tip #64: Start with your fingers, not the vibrator.

A giant noisy vibrator is much like a big penis invading your space—it's a little scary unless you're prepared for it. So try starting with manual finger stimulation to learn anatomy.

You don't have to use a mirror if you're feeling shy, but it is best to do it a bit later, just to understand your own personal body. Pinpoint your clitoris and map out the lips.

Depending on your own comfort level you may bring yourself to a high level of arousal and finish with your hands, or maybe then switch to the vibrator and let it finish the job.

Tip #65: Take it slow, just as a man would take his first sexual encounter slow and with more attention to sensation.

Start using the vibrator on your thighs and proceed to the outer lips and inner lips. Spend time stimulating non-genital parts like breasts, or even the neck, back, buttocks and tailbone. Remember, a full body orgasm usually results from continual stimulation of ALL your body and not just your genitals. Keep the settings slow at first to get used to the texture, sound and feeling.

Remember what we previously discussed about nerve endings in the vagina. Spend time gently moving the vibrator on top of all parts inside your vagina, seeing how it feels. This will give you an idea of what you need during sex with a partner and the intensity and speed necessary.

Tip #66: After moving the vibrator around the vagina's pressure points, it's time to experiment with combination techniques.

For example, you can thrust the vibrator inside like a penis while keeping the pulsation going strong. Or you can stimulate your clit manually while you insert a vibrator deeper inside. You could experiment with timing, and have the rhythmic strokes of penetration coincide with clitoral strokes. You could even use more than one vibrators on a number of erogenous zones—such as clitoral stimulation (pocket rocket), G-spot stimulation ("Rabbit vibrator") and an anal vibrator or nipple teasing toy. Some toys are "double shafted" and let you stimulate part of your vagina while also letting you feel clitoral, anal or G-spot stimulation at the same time.

The Dildo: What's the use of a dildo since it doesn't vibrate? A dildo is typically a more realistic version of a penis, since penises don't "hum" or convulse, and some models even feel real thanks to imitation flesh. They also feel more natural with penetration, especially when combined with generous lubricant.

Tip #67: Practice doing the same with a dildo—letting its "skin" touch you and getting used to the feel of it on your body.

This is what a penis will feel like, more or less, so start experimenting with different ways the penis can interact with your vagina, what speeds, touches and locations work best.

Tip #68: Give yourself a hands free experience with a dildo.

Most of the time you will not be sliding a man's penis into you—you will either let your partner choose a position or you choose a position, one that puts you in greater control. Such as the woman on top position, which is ideal for inducing orgasm by reaching G-spot, A-spot and so on. A hands-free dildo, or even your own set up of a dildo flying on a hair (flat or raised up) can let you learn what it feels like to grind against a penis and see how it feels penetrating you.

Tip #69: Don't forget to experiment with different parts of the "penis", from the sensitive head (which can be rubbed against your clitoris), to the hard shaft that can stimulate multiple parts inside and outside the vulva whether through penetration or even sliding atop.

Size doesn't really matter as you will learn soon enough, since any penis is capable of reaching most erogenous zones inside the vagina, and for the deep spot dildos will suffice nicely.

Learning how to masturbate on your own is not only smart and effective, it's downright "nice"—a nice thing to do to a man who can only move so many mountains, so to speak, when it comes to figuring out how you want it and how you like it. There's no law that says explaining your orgasmic response is required…but a woman who is sex positive and has REAL orgasms, instead of shy, fake ones just to appease a man's ego, is indeed a world of difference. And the vast majority of men definitely prefer real to fake, since they claim they all can tell the difference!

Of course, this is only the first set of lessons in learning how to give and receive great orgasms. Finding the keys to your erotic "Pandora's box" involves another stage, beyond comfort and beyond knowledge. You must go beyond the "ordinary" and predictable sexual routines and boldly go into a new realm of continual discovery. This is known as eroticism—the embracing of what is forbidden.

It's also your secret weapon when finding that awesome orgasm. Let's move on to Chapter 9 and discuss fetishism and eroticism.

Chapter 9: Fetish Sex and Eroticism — To Boldly Go Where Few Men Have Gone Before

Eroticism—simply put, is the difference everyone feels between making love to your spouse the same way you always do, and having hot sex with your current crush against an office wall after work hours. What's "erotic" is oftentimes the opposite of what is normal, reasonable and yes, even what is desired in real life.

In eroticism there is room for fantasy, for living vicariously through novels or movies, and sometimes imagining doing kinky and shameful things we would never do in a world where there are consequences to reckless actions.

Still, exploring the taboo is what fuels your imagination and oftentimes what heightens regular marriage sex (which everyone already has) into the red-hot spicy sex that everyone in the neighborhood envies.

The French philosopher Georges Bataille said it best—"Desire in eroticism is the desire that triumphs over the taboo. It presupposes man in conflict with himself. Eroticism, unlike simple sexual activity, is a psychological quest...eroticism is assenting to life even in death."

Whether you think eroticism as "sin" or evolutionary need (i.e. views of men wanting multiple women to bear their children and women wanting genetically superior children), the one thing you have to agree on is that "illicit sex" always feels more exciting than what you build as your weekly sexual routine.

The Key to Heightening Orgasmic Potential

However, rather than embrace the "psychology" of eroticism, many couples completely avoid it—and unfortunately into common relationship problems like:

- Desire discrepancy or dead bead
- Boredom

- Lack of orgasm or strong orgasm

- Sexual numbness, a lack of passion

- Worst of all, they may even be tempted to cheat—to get that feeling of excitement somewhere else.

But there's no reason to find a mistress or lover just because you want to spice things up. There's no reason to "swing" or have an open marriage just because one or both of you is bored. You can play with eroticism and discover new things about your partner every single time you have sex.

All it takes is communication and the courage to discuss what is taboo.

Tip #70: Resolve to talk with your partner about your unspeakable fantasies, your erotic thoughts, and the stuff you usually avoid saying because of jealousy or fear of judgment.

This is what is called your taboo, your erotic desires deep inside, and what is dying to come out.

One way to do this is to play a sort a game, a sort of sexological improvement of "Truth or

Dare", sometimes called "Would You?" or "May I?" in which both partners review a list of sexual practices with each other, describing how they feel about each one. This is a great idea because most partners are too embarrassed to start confessing their darkest secrets right away. The game makes it a must to at least talk about all these taboo things and how you feel about them. For example, "Definite want to try!" or "Never will try!" or even a "Maybe someday."

You make it a point to try the practices that you might agree with and maybe discuss compromises on the things that you don't want to try.

For example, a common fantasy is in cheating with someone else. It's not going to happen in the real world, but what kind of hot fantasy could be created from this taboo?

Perhaps:

- Watching porn or reading erotica together

- Describing your fantasy or having your partner describe a fantasy of another person

- Roleplaying a scenario involving two lovers meeting each other

The point is, if you work in the "taboo element" into your regular sex sessions, you will definitely see a more profound orgasm in the female partner, who needs that mental fuel to go over the edge. We already discussed that orgasming starts as a mental process, and if you're embracing what already turns her on in idea, then you're HALF WAY there before you place the first kiss! By all means, exploit these taboos and find out what her secret desire is and give her a scenario, an idea or at least a feeling of eroticism. There is always greater joy in giving. So strive to please physically AND mentally.

Tip #71: Try something new every time you have sex, from our list of sexual taboos.

- Roleplaying

- Cheating

- Threesomes or orgies

- Sex with a stranger

- Sex with a friend or coworker
- Bondage and control
- Dominating the other partner
- Causing a little bit of pain with pleasure (i.e. candle wax or spankings)
- Surrendering to the desires of your partner
- Dirty talking
- Being seduced
- Forced fantasies
- Being watched by others while you have sex
- Watching others have sex
- Gender reversals or even gender role play
- Humiliation
- Focus on parts of the body (i.e. butts, feet, armpits, etc.)

- Wearing costumes or even BDSM-style rubber and latex

- Breast milk

- Piercings and tattooing

- Transvestitism

- Swinging or cuckolding

And of course there are many other extremes, and subcategories within each fetish. It's important to remember though, that eroticism is not simply doing what everyone else is doing or doing what you think your partner wants from you. In fact, that's a sure recipe for disaster—doing what you don't like just to please your partner. It will create negative feelings when sex should be only about joy and pleasure!

The key is in, once again, LEARNING YOURSELF.

Fetishism and BDSM

Fetishism and BDSM have gotten a bad rap as of late, with people thinking that it's all about dominance or abusing their partner. It's not—and frankly, it's not just about tying someone up or whipping them or acting all "dominant" or "submissive."

At the root of fetishism is the unique perspective and desires of the individual. While statistically speaking, men have more fetishes than women, it's important to realize that as recently as 100 years ago, women were not expected to have fetishes or kinks, or any real pleasure from sex besides pleasing a man. So give women some time to get in touch with their inner kink. And as always, be supportive when she finally confides.

Tip #72: Be interested, aroused and excited when she shares a "forbidden fantasy."

She might be shy and expecting you to scoff, laugh or judge her for something. Let her know that you find the idea just as sexy and want to recreate it somehow, in a comfortable way you can both agree on.

Alfred Binet, a French psychologist, was among the first to determine that fetishism is the result of associations, and that most if not all fetishes came from an object or experience in childhood, oftentimes involving trauma. It's not uncommon that women who were terrified of being spanked as a child, develop spanking fetishes.

So yes, finding these fetishes could take some work, especially if your partner is shy and typically doesn't open up about past sexual experiences in general. This is why talking about other people's fetishes, for example "what you heard" a friend does, or has done, etc. These are nice and easy segues into discussing what your sex life COULD be, if only you wanted to discuss it openly. Who knows, maybe talking about all these crazy things other people do, may jog your partner's memory and she may remember something from her past that turned her on greatly. That's some extra "fuel" you can use to achieve a greater-than-average mental orgasm.

Mental arousal for a woman is like the fuel that runs the engine. Don't go by "fumes" or just mechanical sexual performance alone. It's not about the "how hard" you penetrate…it's always about the "why." Welcome to the female mind!

BDSM and taboos are scary topics for first-timers, which brings us up to another important point—the obligation to be kind and conscientious when being with your lover.

Forget everything you learned about BDSM from the media. Being nice really works and here's why…

Chapter 10: How to be a Considerate Lover

Make no mistake about it—being nice means everything in sex. No, it's not going to do you a lot of favors in dating, but that's not where we're at. We're at that delicate point where self-doubt is devastating, where judgment is cruel, and where the look on your face and tone in your voice means EVERYTHING.

You do have to be nice because your partner is counting on you to create a safe environment for her, one where she won't be humiliated, won't have her feelings hurts, and won't be scared at your enthusiastic "in character" performance for all that fetishistic roleplaying you want to try.

This brings us to:

Tip #73: Always have a safe word if you're going to kink it up.

This means a special word your partner uses to let you know things are going too far and it's time to take it back a notch. More importantly, be attentive to her so you can tell if she's becoming worried, scared or uncomfortable but is not quite saying it yet.

The current media craze with *Fifty Shades of Grey* is somewhat misleading, considering that the book promotes antagonizing your submissive partner and dominating her at all cost. This isn't the true philosophy of BDSM or consensual fetishism and discipline.

In the "real thing," the submissive is the one that wants to be disciplined, dominated and controlled. Usually, the submissive knows exactly what he or she wants and finds a "master" or "dominant" that understands the consensual psychology of the BDSM lifestyle. The dominant is in control for the sake of roleplaying; but the submissive always has the right to change the dynamic if she becomes scared, hurt, or edgy.

Always play it safe by being the conscientious partner, the one who only gives your partner what she wants.

Tip #74: Do NOT ever take unjustified risks like:

- Forcing a sex act on your partner she might not like or that you haven't even discussed yet

- Ignoring her if she says something hurts or feels strange and uncomfortable

- Demanding sex when she clearly is not in the mood

- Being "dominant" even if your submissive doesn't feel like playing

- Pushing your fantasies on your partner, especially if she is not feeling excited about it

And the reason for this is not because "you should be nice," not just that—it's because you're going to not only miss out on the big explosive orgasms you want her to have, but you're also going to sabotage future orgasms and perhaps your whole relationship, since you're ignoring her needs and wants and are associating sex with NEGATIVE EMOTIONS.

How to be a Dominant Lover or a Horny Submissive

Now all that said, there are clearly roles to play in the sexual relationship, and these roles seem recurring.

- Men should be strong, confident
- Women should be submissive, "seduced" and desired by the stronger male

We're not getting into the sexual politics or into the genetic or social argumentation of equal rights. It's simply a matter of common sense. In order for a woman to feel instinctively attracted to a man, he must be confident, sure of what he wants (her!) and comfortable with the sexual experience.

Tip #75: The way you feel inside should be expressed outwardly, namely in:

- Speaking clearly and in a firm voice
- Keeping strong eye contact
- Smiling and giving signs of your approval, not constantly scowling

- Having the confidence to get naked and to undress her

- Being the "seducer" and not the one waiting to be seduced

- Using confident terminology for body parts, previously agreed upon. (Many women have no problem with dirty talking, but some might...it's best to discuss this beforehand)

- A man KNOWS her body. He doesn't have to ask what to do next.

Of course, with gender reversals it is sometimes common to see a woman seducing a man and him playing the submissive. But in the majority of cases, the man must present himself as a confident lover, completely sure of what he wants.

Tip #76: Get reassurances and establish boundaries.

The instinct of man is to ask his lover, "How am I doing?" but that doesn't sound confident in the context of taboo sex. Instead, get her reassurances that it feels good with your yes or no questions converted into sexy or dirty talk. For instance, "Tell me you like the way my penis feels…" He's asking permission and getting reassurance here, but dressing it up so as not to break character in his dominant role.

Equally important is established boundaries EARLY ON, before taboo or BDSM sex even happens. The worst thing you can do is to "surprise" a woman by doing something she doesn't like. This is why communication beforehand is essential. Discuss not only what is a "yes" or a "maybe" but also what is a "No" and why it's a No. Take her boundaries seriously and don't try to change her mind as this only causes stress—and as we know, stress and negative association is the antidote to really good orgasms.

Sometimes being a good lover is just a matter of avoiding the most common mistakes, and making "all the right moves." You might be surprised at how easy it is to be a "sex god" for your partner, and all because you actually listened to what she said, sensed what she wanted, and did NOT do something stupid…

Stupid mistakes, which were going to discuss in Chapter 11.

Chapter 11: The Most Common Mistakes Guys Make in Bed

Oftentimes knowing what most guys are doing wrong will help YOU to stay a class above them. It's not only about sensing what a woman wants. Sometimes a man's instincts are off, and that's when it's time to consult a list of DO NOTs, to make sure you're not making the same common mistake as every other frustrated lover.

DO NOT: Think that she's going to have sex with you, anywhere, anytime just like in the movies.

Tip #77: Spend more time creating a romantic, safe and arousing scene.

Setting means everything for a woman who's trying to find a comfort zone to start her mental orgasmic process.

DO NOT: Rush after the genitals. Yes, we know you're all excited to try our clit, G-spot and A-spot techniques, but for now…

Tip #78: Don't skimp on foreplay.

Remember your Tantra and Sensate Focus code of honor: don't even start arousing her genitals until you've made her come once just from paying attention to the rest of her body. That's why it's called a FULL BODY orgasm! Move slow. It's much better to hear her say, "Hurry and screw me!" then it is to hear, "Whoah, slow down!" If you're in a hurry for ANY REASON, it's not the right time to do this.

DO NOT: Ignore her body language thinking your sexual strategy is foolproof.

Tip #79: Always pay attention to her body, how it moves; how her voice sounds, what she is saying, and what she is NOT responding too.

Too many guys make the mistake of thinking they can make her come with their great new moves, rather than adapting to the unique sexual experiences and improvising according to her wants.

DO NOT: Pout, throw a hissy fit or get agitated because things are not working out as you imagined.

Tip #80: Be cool. Be strong. Be dominant and in control.

It doesn't matter if she laughs, or if she's doing something annoying (perhaps even telling you what she doesn't like or rejecting your fantasy, etc.), or if she tells you the G-spot move is not working. You have to laugh it off and go along with it…or else you'll upset her mood and have to start back at square one. She is in control of the orgasm, always remember this.

DO NOT: Think she's going to act like a porn star just to please you. Through no choice of her own, she's not going to—she probably doesn't even know what porn girls act like. She doesn't want to be disrespected. She's not going to overact. She's not going to figure out that you like it dirty and rough. A lot of your fantasy fulfillment should be negotiated beforehand to avoid misunderstandings. She might not even be inclined to do certain things, so don't be too disappointed if she vetoes some items on your list. This is real sex, not like as depicted on TV!

Tip #81: Learn her reactions and embrace her unique style of orgasming.

Don't manipulate her into being someone else, when what you ultimately want is HER, being herself...and coming like a fountain.

DO NOT: Be content with making her orgasm just once. Or demanding she have multiples every time.

Tip #82: Communicate and let her decide.

She may want more than one orgasm and if so, give it to her in just the way she wants it. Or, she may feel more satisfied with one long and intense orgasm, and not want to come multiple times. Either way is fine, and she's the most qualified to decide how much is enough.

Thus far, we've covered a lot of information for helping women to get in touch with their sexuality, and helping men learn sexual techniques that are sure to work, with the right environment and attitude.

Now for the bad news. Sometimes it's not enough. Sometimes your partner is just NOT going to orgasm, whether you scream to the moon, pound her for hours on end, or tongue flick until you get lock-jaw.

The good news is that even if she has problems with anorgasmia, there is always a solution to try. Let's review our final chapter.

Chapter 12: Cures for Performance Anxiety and Anorgasmia

Anorgasmia, the inability to orgasm, can be a temporary problem or even a long-term issue that requires medical attention. Much like erectile dysfunction, it is best to analyze the problem and try to determine if there is a psychological problem that could explain it, before making it a medical issue.

The first thing to determine is whether your partner's anorgasmia is one of pain (sex is literally too painful, because of a constricted vagina) or she is simply not getting wet enough, or maybe she is getting wet and excited, but still cannot orgasm.

Obviously painful intercourse or dyspareunia requires some medical attention.

Tip #83: If sex is painful, a doctor could advise you to seek:

- Surgery
- Medications (such as Osphena)
- Desensitization therapy (i.e. pelvic crunches, partial entry over a period of time

Tip #84: If the problem is psychological or there is no particular physical element, couples counseling, psychotherapy (usually for major psychological issues beyond sex) or sex therapy may be recommended.

Many cases of anorgasmia are actually caused by relationship difficulties, including lack of trust, or past trauma, or unresolved issues with the partner.

Tip #85: For low libido or for an improperly functioning vagina (i.e. dryness or lack of sexual response), hormone replacement therapy may be the best solution, speaking of estrogen therapy or even testosterone therapy.

One remarkable achievement in modern sex therapy treatment has been the invention of the Eros-Clitoral Therapy Device, a device invented solely for the purpose of addressing female sexual arousal disorder (FSAD). The small vacuum device bringing the clitoris out for greater stimulation is to be used over a period of six weeks, and has shown good results in improved lubrication, orgasmic response and overall sexual satisfaction.

Tip #86: Invest in your mental and physical health.

A healthy diet and exercise actually do work wonders for a woman's sex life and may be a contributing cause towards sexual fulfillment if she is in bad health.

In addition to all essential vitamins, some herbal substances like Zestra (oil) and Argin-Max (a supplement) have shown positive results in helping to improve clitoral stimulation and the capacity to feel arousal, oftentimes through the improvement of blood flow to the vagina.

Tip #87: Get a little extra help from hypnosis.

Much of anorgasmia related issues stem from relationship problems, or childhood trauma, or sometimes even anxiety. Listening to calming and self-affirming hypnosis on disc or MP3 can help you to refocus your thoughts and feelings on positive imagery and emotions, thereby slowly but surely changing the way your mind works—and builds up orgasmic resistance.

Yes the solution to every sexual problem, and psychological issue for that matter, is to focus more effort on reprogramming your brain (and your partner's brain) with positive imagery, affirming thoughts and good associations.

That's wonderful news because that means even if you've messed up before and caused a partner to become reclusive or uninterested in sex, you can still make things right. You can rekindle the relationship by honestly communicating, taking small and slow steps towards creating intimacy, and this time, approaching sex from a more educated view.

It's never too late to try. It's never too late, nor shall it ever be too late, to please your partner and give her one amazing night to remember.

Conclusion

We live in an age where we have so much information it's almost overkill; not everyone understands the best sources for this information and ends up just as uneducated as if there was no information available. Most important of all is gaining a medical, clinical and sexological understanding of orgasmic response coming from trusted industry sources.

We don't need an expert telling us that "all women squirt because of a secret G-spot move that works every time." That's the sensational type of sex edu-tainment that may cause more problems than it solves. What we've learned over the course of these chapters is that orgasmic sex is very much an individual process, one that couples really have to explore together.

Yes, an understanding anatomy is helpful but in the end, communication is the only thing that's going to work and give your partner the best orgasms ever. It takes two to tango, because they have to work in unison, much like a dance, where each partner knows his or her "choreography" and then the two mesh perfectly together, totally responsive to the other's needs as if by instinct.

None of it is instinct or luck though—it's just consistent practice and the determination to be a good lover. The orgasm isn't a mystery of the body. It's a mystery of the mind and it's a mystery you can solve, along with your partner. But this is the kind of enjoyable research that you don't mind staying up late to do.

Printed in Great Britain
by Amazon